The Radiant Skin

Diet

I0424545

The Best Ways to Incorporate Anti -
Aging Food Ingredients into your Diet

BY: SOPHIA FREEMAN

© 2019 Sophia Freeman All Rights Reserved

COPYRIGHTED

Liability

This publication is meant as an informational tool. The individual purchaser accepts all liability if damages occur because of following the directions or guidelines set out in this publication. The Author bears no responsibility for reparations caused by the misuse or misinterpretation of the content.

Copyright

The content of this publication is solely for entertainment purposes and is meant to be purchased by one individual. Permission is not given to any individual who copies, sells or distributes parts or the whole of this publication unless it is explicitly given by the Author in writing.

My gift to you!

Thank you, cherished reader, for purchasing my book and taking the time to read it. As a special reward for your decision, I would like to offer a gift of free and discounted books directly to your inbox. All you need to do is fill in the box below with your email address and name to start getting amazing offers in the comfort of your own home. You will never miss an offer because a reminder will be sent to you. Never miss a deal and get great deals without having to leave the house! Subscribe now and start saving!

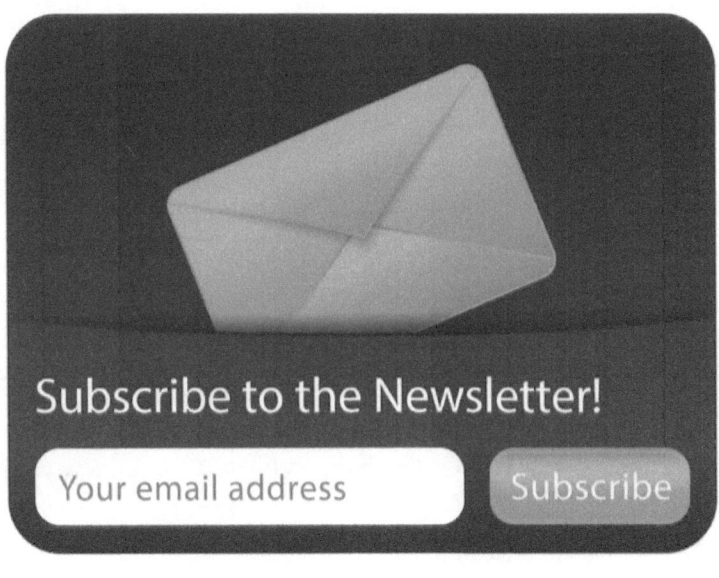

* * * * ★ ★ ★ ★ * * *

Table of Contents

Anti-Aging Food Recipes

zzzzzzzzzzzzzzzzzzzzzzzzzzzzzzzzzzzzzzzzzzzzzzzzzzzzzzzzzzzzzzzzz

1) Carrot and Bacon Casserole

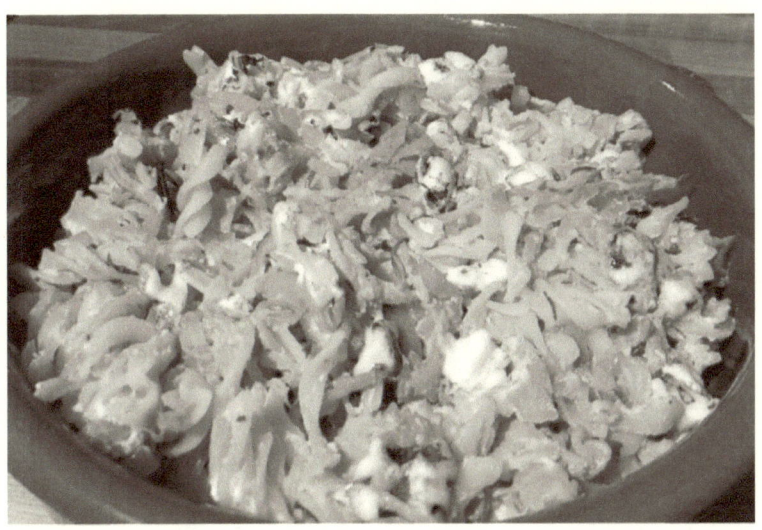

Carrots have been associated with great vision for many years. While this is true, they have other exceptional properties it's important to mention here. The carrots contain nutrients which help your skin cell damage repairs and also help protect your skin from being damaged from sun exposure long term. Enjoy this special casserole we have created with carrots, especially for you!

Ingredient List:

- 3 medium shredded carrots
- 1 shredded zucchini
- 3 minced cloves garlic
- 1 medium chopped sweet onion
- 6 thick slices Smoked Applewood bacon
- ¼ c. honey
- Salt, pepper to taste
- 3 tablespoons chopped fresh parsley
- 2 tablespoons unsalted butter

Serving Size: 4-6

Cooking Time: 55 minutes

zzzzzzzzzzzzzzzzzzzzzzzzzzzzzzzzzzzzzzzzzzzzzzzzzzzzzzzzzzzzzzzz

Instructions:

1. Preheat the oven to 400 degrees F. Grease and set aside a square baking pan.
2. Cook the bacon in a skillet until crispy, but don't overcook.
3. Keep the bacon grease in the skillet and remove the cooked bacon.
4. Cook the garlic, onion, the zucchini and carrots in the bacon grease. Add a little butter if necessary and salt/pepper.
5. Once the veggies are cooked place them in the dish and also add the crumbled pieces of bacon.
6. Add the honey all over and the chopped fresh parsley.
7. Bake in the oven for 30 minutes.

2) Simple Olive Oil Pasta

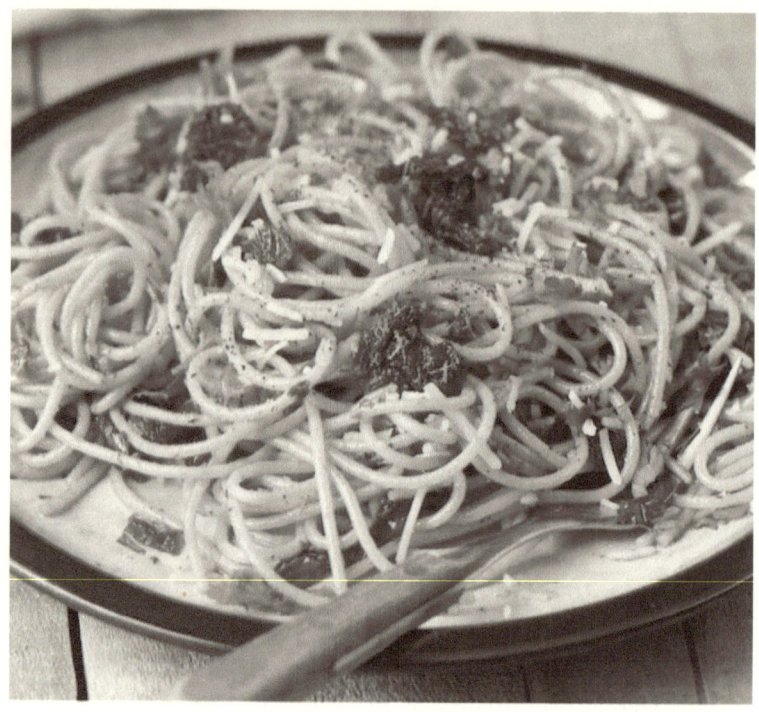

I think most households now have a bottle of olive oil sitting in the pantry. Not only can you use it to cook your veggies, your meats and other foods, but you can make some awesome sauces or vinaigrettes. The polyphenols included in this type of oil are powerful, full of antioxidants. The omega 3 fatty acids it contains, is full of HDL or good cholesterol, and can certainly benefit you in many ways, including anti-aging and skin health.

Ingredient List:

- 1 box or package angel hair pasta
- ¼ c. olive oil
- 6 minced cloves garlic
- 2 c. chopped spinach
- 1 c. shredded Mozzarella cheese
- Salt, black pepper to taste

Serving Size: 4

Cooking Time: 35 minutes

zzzzzzzzzzzzzzzzzzzzzzzzzzzzzzzzzzzzzzzzzzzzzzzzzzzzzzzzzzzzzzz

Instructions:

1. Cook the pasta as indicated on the package. Drain and set aside.
2. In a large saucepan, heat a little olive oil and cook the garlic for 5 minutes.
3. Add the spinach, salt, pepper and cook another 5 minutes.
4. Add the rest of the oil with the cooked pasta and the mozzarella cheese.
5. Combine really well and keep warm until the Mozzarella cheese is all melted.
6. Serve
7. Many additional toppings or ingredients can be used, such as sundried tomatoes, mushrooms and others. Find your favorite oily pasta dish and stick with it!

3) Garlicky Chicken Soup

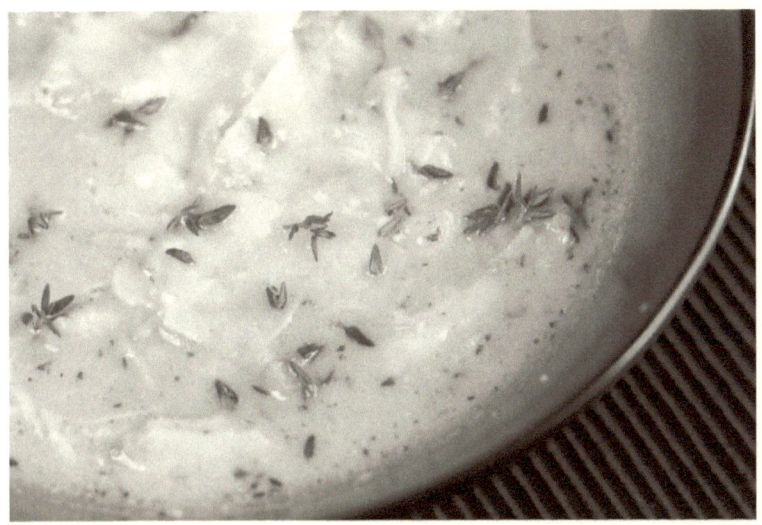

My mother used to tell me to take a bite of fresh garlic clove if I was fighting a cold. She was partially right, because it does help prevent infections, but she did not warn me about the strong breath for days to come! So, I prefer now to use cooked garlic or minced garlic at least in my recipe, such as this one below. However, I learned since then that garlic also has amazing anti-aging properties: it will help you prevent wrinkles on your skin just as much as zinc and selenium do.

Ingredient List:

- 10 minced cloves garlic
- 2 tablespoons unsalted butter
- 1 large sliced yellow onion
- 6 c. chicken broth
- 2 c. shredded chicken
- 1 tablespoon chopped fresh thyme
- 1 tablespoon chopped fresh oregano
- Salt, pepper to taste

Serving Size: 4-6

Cooking Time: 45 minutes

zzzzzzzzzzzzzzzzzzzzzzzzzzzzzzzzzzzzzzzzzzzzzzzzzzzzzzzzzzzzzz

Instructions:

1. Brown the garlic in a large saucepan, using butter.
2. Add the yellow onion next and let it cook for another 10 minutes.
3. Finally pour the chicken broth, stir and add the fresh herbs as well as salt, and pepper.
4. Add the cooked chicken and adjust any seasonings you might think needs it.
5. Enjoy especially on a winter day!

4) Braised Orange Chicken

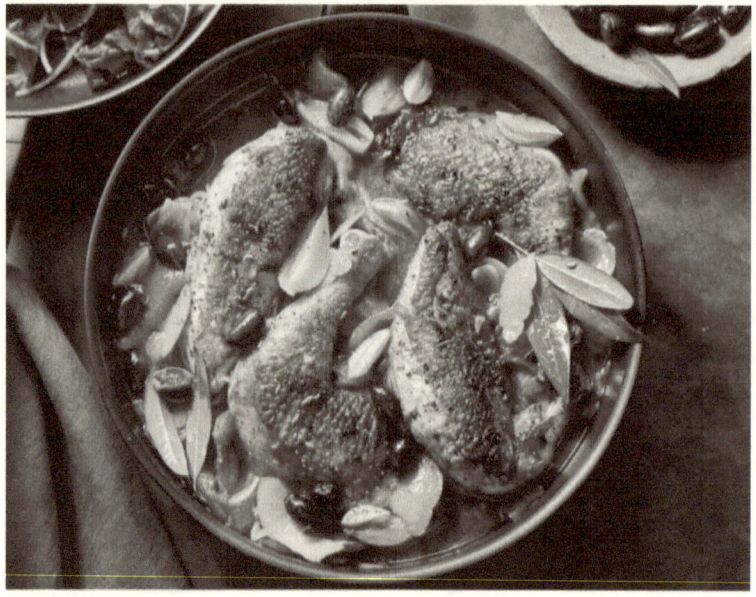

We sometimes forget to incorporate oranges into our dishes at times when they could add so much flavor and so many health benefits. Oranges can help you fight aging because they are full of water and will help hydrate your skin. They also offer a lot of Vitamin C to your body which helps you in all kinds of ways.

Ingredient List:

- 4 skinless chicken breasts
- 2 tablespoons olive oil
- 2 sliced oranges
- 1 sliced lemon
- salt, pepper to taste
- small bunch fresh thyme sprigs
- 2 tablespoons chopped fresh basil
- 2 cups chicken broth
- ½ cup orange juice
- 3 tablespoons brown sugar
- ½ cup dry white wine

Serving Size: 12+

Cooking Time: 45 minutes

zzzzzzzzzzzzzzzzzzzzzzzzzzzzzzzzzzzzzzzzzzzzzzzzzzzzzzzzzzzzzz

Instructions:

1. Preheat the oven to 375 degrees F.
2. In a large skillet, heat the olive oil. After seasoning with salt and pepper, brown the chicken for a few minutes on each side.
3. Place the chicken breasts in large greased baking pan next.
4. Keep the oil in the skillet and deglaze with the wine, adding also the orange juice and brown sugar.
5. Pour this wine mixture on the chicken and add the chicken broth as well.
6. Place the thyme on top of the chicken as well as the orange and lemon slices.
7. Bake in the oven for about 45 minutes to 50 minutes.
8. Serve on a rice bed with the oranges.

5) Stuffed Strawberries

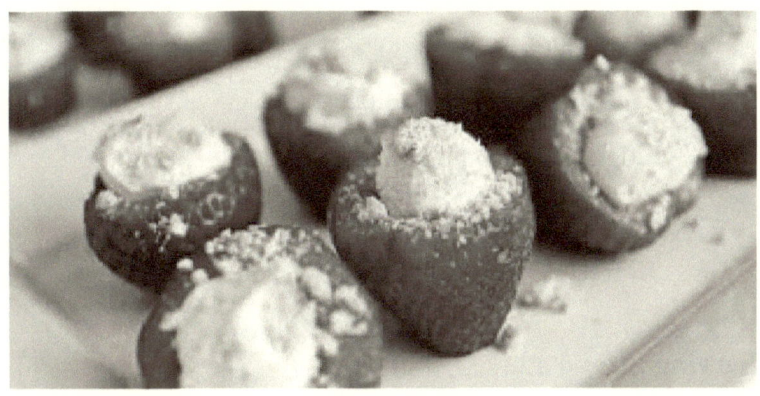

Strawberries are taking the stage here and we are proposing a quite fun and delicious recipe to add to your collection. Know that strawberries have these specific properties: reduce inflammation, help health of your bones, high blood pressure natural medicine, and help overall build very strong and healthy hair and nails. Also, let's mention that one full cup of strawberries contains less than 45 calories, perfect for any diet.

Ingredient List:

- 1 package cream cheese (softened)
- 3 tablespoons maple syrup
- 2 tablespoons brown sugar
- Pinch cinnamon
- ¼ c. granola cereals
- 36 fresh strawberries

Serving Size: 6-12

Cooking Time: 50 minutes

zzzzzzzzzzzzzzzzzzzzzzzzzzzzzzzzzzzzzzzzzzzzzzzzzzzzzzzzzzzzzzzz

Instructions:

1. Wash and prepare all strawberries by removing a little of the core.
2. In a bowl, mix the cream cheese, the maple syrup, brown sugar and cinnamon.
3. Stuff each strawberry with a generous portion of the cream cheese mixture.
4. Place the strawberries on a serving plate and sprinkle with granola mix.
5. If you prefer other toppings, you could very well sprinkle some shredded chocolate or roasted shredded coconut.

6) Brussel Sprouts Fun Skewers

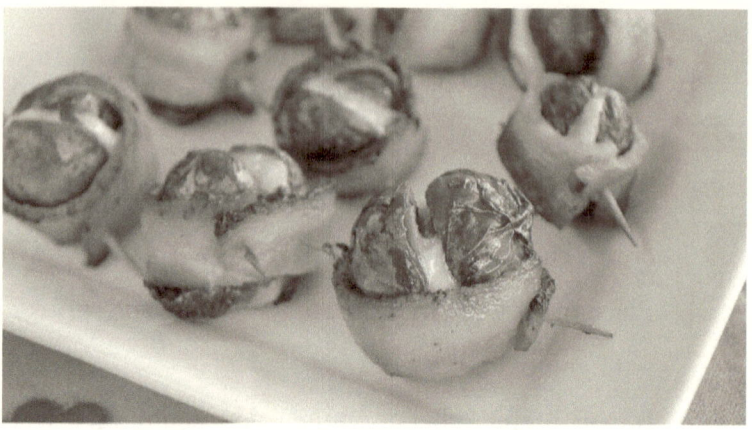

Brussel sprouts are definitely one of the veggies that people usually either love or hate. Marrying this nutrient-dense veggie with bacon can help many get used to the taste, especially your skeptical children. Brussel sprouts are full of vitamin A and C as well as folate, promoting the production of collagen, and keeping your skin elasticity top notch.

Ingredient List:

- 1-pound maple flavored turkey bacon
- 2 pounds fresh Brussels sprouts
- ¼ c. maple syrup
- 1 teaspoon onion powder
- Salt, pepper to taste
- Skewers (wooden or metal)

Serving Size: 12+

Cooking Time: 45 minutes

zzzzzzzzzzzzzzzzzzzzzzzzzzzzzzzzzzzzzzzzzzzzzzzzzzzzzzzzzzzzzzz

Instructions:

1. Preheat the oven to 400 degrees.
2. Set aside a greased baking sheet.
3. In a large saucepan, boil the water with salt. Cook the brussel sprouts for about 10 minute or so and let them drain well.
4. In a skillet, cook the bacon for 5-7 minutes. This will only precook it. Cut in the bacon into 3 equal pieces.
5. Mix the maple syrup with the salt, pepper and onion powder in a small bowl.
6. Start assembling the skewers by using one Brussel sprout, one piece of bacon and so on.
7. Generously brush the maple syrup mixture on each skewer.
8. Line them up on the baking sheet and cook for 20 minutes or so.
9. Serve with or without a dipping sauce.

7) Wild Orzo and Mushrooms

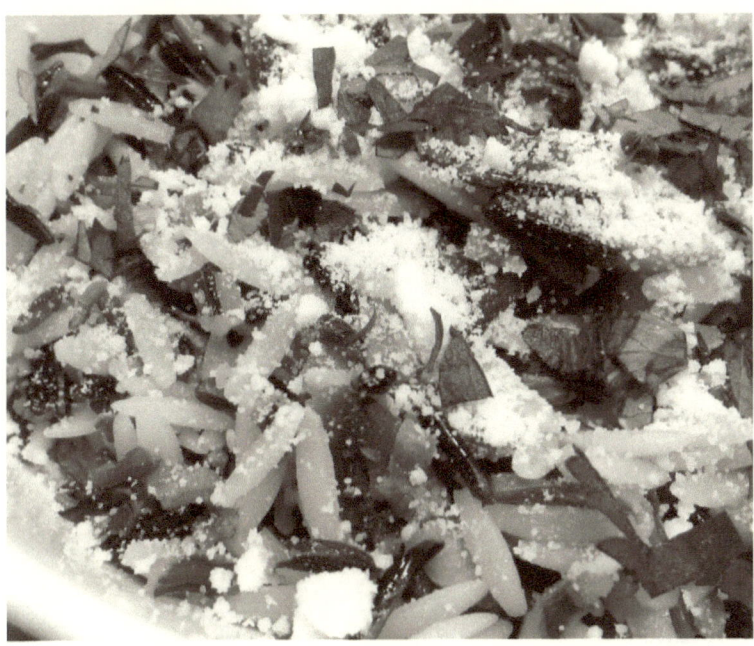

Mushrooms are so tasty prepared in many different ways. My son prefers them sautéed and placed on top of his burger. I love mushroom soups. But this recipe below is also a winner in my book! Also, keep in mind the health benefits you get from these fungi. You will be possibly surprised to learn that mushrooms can help beautify your skin. They have awesome anti-inflammatory value and can also clear up any toxins you cumulate against your will.

Ingredient List:

- 3 c. beef broth
- 1 ½ c. uncooked orzo
- 2 c. sliced shiitake mushrooms
- 1 c. dry red wine
- 3 minced cloves garlic
- 2 minced onions
- 2 tablespoons olive oil
- Salt, pepper to taste
- ½ c. shredded Gouda cheese

Serving Size: 4

Cooking Time: 45 minutes

zzzzzzzzzzzzzzzzzzzzzzzzzzzzzzzzzzzzzzzzzzzzzzzzzzzzzzzzzzzzzzzzzz

Instructions:

1. Boil the beef broth and cook the orzo.
2. Meanwhile, sauté the garlic, onions and mushrooms in olive oil, salt, and pepper.
3. When both veggies are cooked and orzo ready, combine in a skillet and add the red wine, let is reduced.
4. Finally, add the Gouda cheese and let it simmer until the cheese is melted.
5. Serve and enjoy this delicious side dish!

8) Sugary Grapes

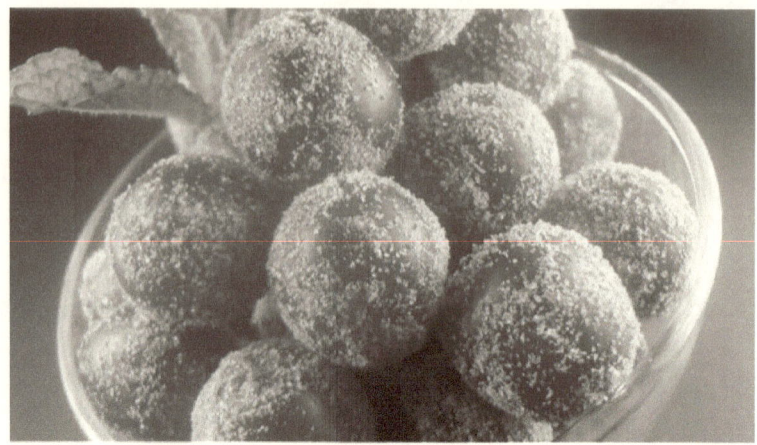

Sure, you can choose to eat grapes as-is, they are yummy enough and juicy enough. But this recipe will change things up just a little bit. Grapes will help reduce inflammation in your body and keep you from aging quickly. Also, it will help you fight the bad effects of the sun damage on your skin, which is rather important. So, eat these grapes up!

Ingredient List:

- Bunch of seedless grapes, about 50
- 1 package gelatin mix
- ½ cup coconut palm sugar

Serving Size: 4-6

Cooking Time: 1 hour +

ZZZZZZZZZZZZZZZZZZZZZZZZZZZZZZZZZZZZZZZZZZZZZZZZZZZZZZZZZZZZ

Instructions:

1. You can choose either red or green seedless grapes, it does not matter. Make sure you do wash them carefully and drain any water.
2. Next, prepare the gelatin. Sprinkle it into place and let it sit.
3. Coat each grape with the gelatin mixture.
4. In a different plate place the coconut palm sugar and repeat the same, but coating again.
5. That's it! You now have pretty sugary grapes to snack on.
6. Refrigerate until ready to serve.

9) Yogurt, Nut and Pumpkin Dessert Cup

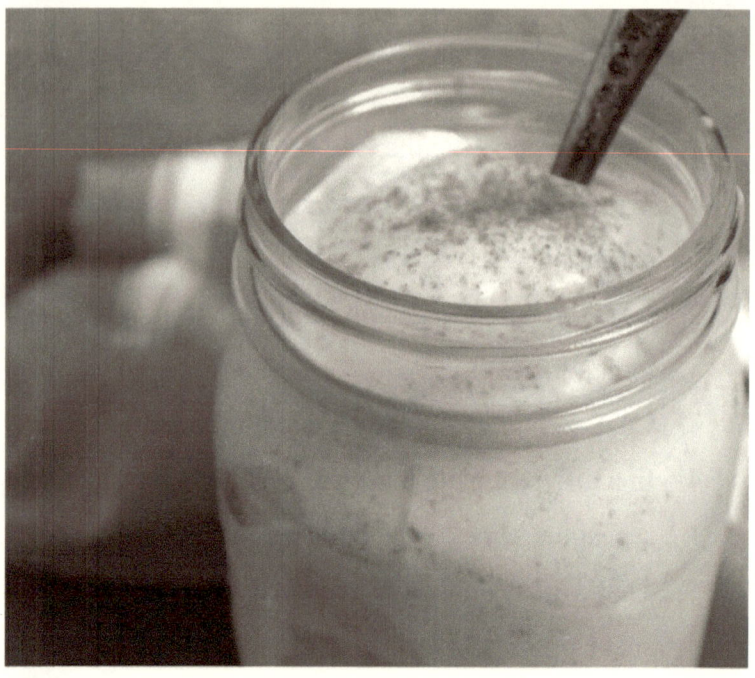

Although it might not be the ultimate anti-aging food, yogurt does have a variety of valuable properties that are worth mentioning and make it a very important food item to include in your diet. Because yogurt offers good bacteria, it does help your gut, or your intestinal system to stay healthy longer and help you look and feel better.

Try this recipe below; you won't even think you are simply eating yogurt, because it is so tasty.

Ingredient List:

- 2 c. Greek plain yogurt
- 1 can pumpkin puree
- 3 tablespoons maple syrup
- 1 teaspoon cinnamon
- Pinch nutmeg
- 1 teaspoon vanilla extract
- 2 c. whipped cream
- Chopped nuts as toppings

Serving Size: 4

Cooking Time: 1 hour

zzzzzzzzzzzzzzzzzzzzzzzzzzzzzzzzzzzzzzzzzzzzzzzzzzzzzzzzzzzzz

Instructions:

1. In a large mixing bowl, mix the yogurt and the pumpkin puree, the maple syrup, cinnamon and nutmeg with an electric mixer.
2. In a different bowl, mix together the whipped cream and vanilla extract.
3. Refrigerate both mixtures for an hour.
4. After 30 minutes, combine both mixtures well.
5. Divide the mixture in 4 serving cups; add some nuts as topping before serving.
6. Keep the cups in the refrigerator until you are ready to serve.

10) Beet Bites

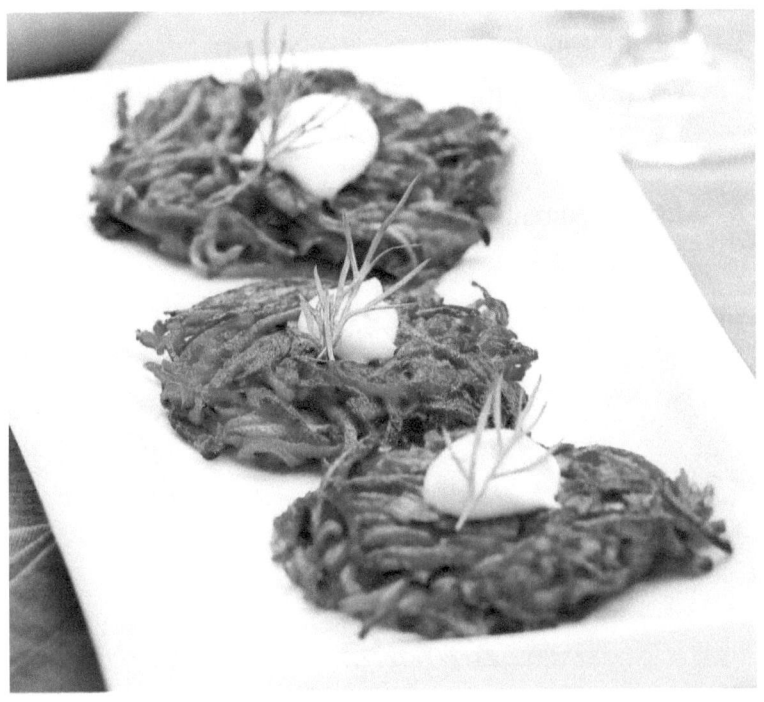

Beets are not a greatly popular root vegetable. They can be quite bitter if not prepared with other ingredients. This recipe will help you appreciate beets all over again. Meanwhile, be aware that they can provide you some amazing anti-aging properties for your skin, but also your health, brain and vision. The carotenoids, fibers and antioxidants will help your eyes stay healthier longer and your brain and heart stronger.

Ingredient List:

- 4 medium grated beets
- 2 minced green onions
- ¼ c. tapioca flour
- 1 egg
- 2 tablespoons whole milk
- Salt, pepper to taste
- 1 tablespoon sweet paprika
- 2 tablespoons avocado oil or olive oil

Serving Size: 4-6

Cooking Time: 45 minutes

zzzzzzzzzzzzzzzzzzzzzzzzzzzzzzzzzzzzzzzzzzzzzzzzzzzzzzzzzzzzzzz

Instructions:

1. Trim, wash, and peel all beets first.
2. Then, grate them as fine as you can over a large mixing bowl.
3. Remember, you are making a type of pancake, but with beets, so be mindful of the texture you want to obtain.
4. Heat the oil in a skillet and cook the beets with salt and pepper for about 10 minutes. Add the green onions also for another 5 minutes.
5. Stir often so nothing sticks. Remove from the heat and place back into a large mixing bowl.
6. Add the tapioca flour, the milk and egg. Combine well and pour the batter, once pancake at a time in the skillet again.
7. You will most have to add a little more oil to do so.
8. Flip the beet pancake after 5 minutes on one side. You want it to be a nice golden and red color.
9. Serve with your favorite toppings; maple syrup, honey, agave syrup or even yoghurt or sour cream.

11) Lemon and Herb Grilled Salmon Filets

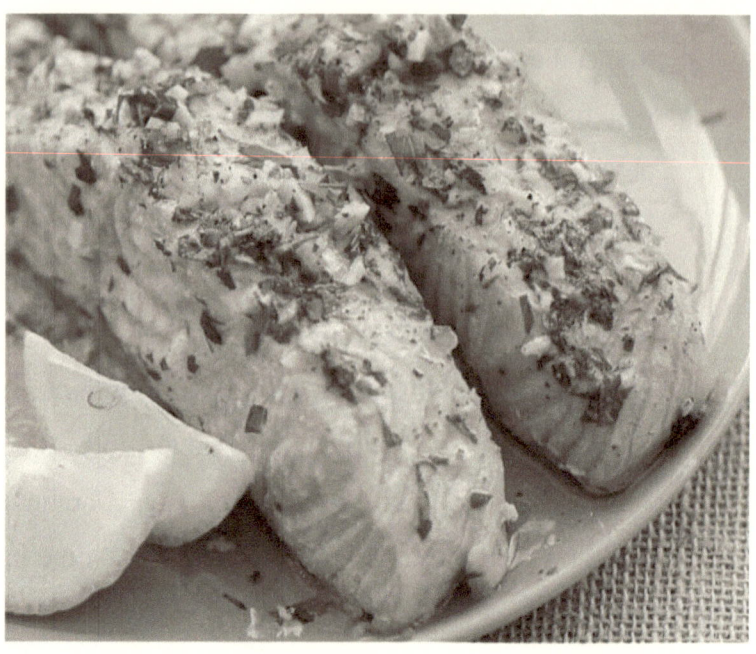

We talk about the importance of eating oily fish, such as salmon all the time, but why is that exactly? Well, these types of fish offer what we call omega 3 fatty acids to your body. It has been proven that skin cancer and many health complications can be prevented by consuming a regular amount of omega 3s. So, go ahead and make this recipe tomorrow night, it's delicious and so good for you!

Ingredient List:

- 4 salmon filets
- ¼ c. olive oil
- 2 tablespoons fresh chopped cilantro
- 2 tablespoons fresh chopped parsley
- 2 tablespoons fresh chopped basil
- 3 tablespoons lime juice
- 1 tablespoon lime zest
- Salt, black pepper to taste
- 1 tablespoon chili powder

Serving Size: 4

Cooking Time: 1 hour +

zzzzzzzzzzzzzzzzzzzzzzzzzzzzzzzzzzzzzzzzzzzzzzzzzzzzzzzzzzzzzz

Instructions:

1. Preheat the oven to 400 degrees. You could very well grill these awesome filets, but it's up to you. If you chose to do so, just turn on the grill now.
2. Grease a large rectangular pan and set aside.
3. In a medium mixing bowl, place the oil and add the cilantro, basil, parsley, lime juice, lime zest, chili powder and salt/pepper.
4. Whisk all ingredients for marinade well.
5. Clean and season all salmon filets and then place them skin down in the pan.
6. Brush carefully and generously each filet with the dressing.
7. Bake in the oven for 25 minutes or so or until you are certain that the salmon is well cooked.

12) Spinach and Bean Salad

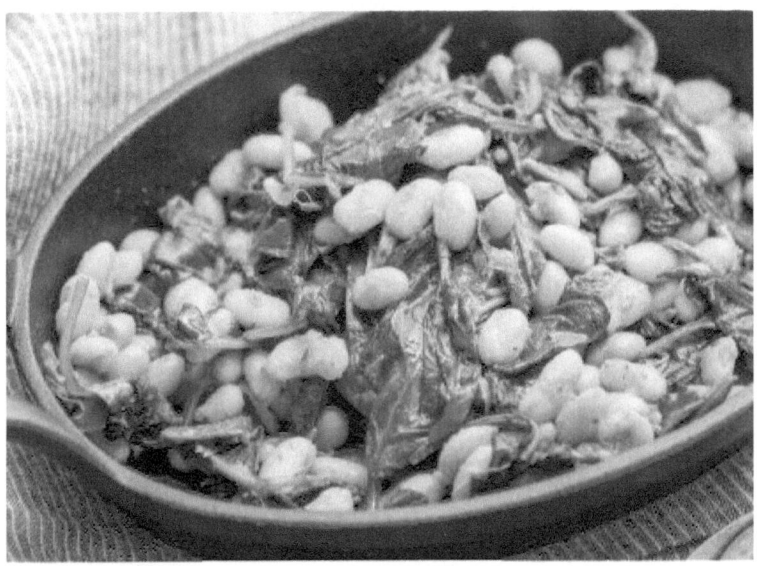

I am a spinach lover, so eating it is certainly not a chore or punishment for me. I can eat them in a salad, as a raw veggie with or without dip, sautéed with garlic or even added to a casserole. Spinach offers many health benefits, including of course what this book is all about, anti-aging ones. The zeaxanthin and lutein, specific antioxidants contained in this green leafed veggie, are responsible for helping to keep your skin protected from ultraviolet rays and looking young.

Ingredient List:

- 4 c. fresh spinach chopped
- 3 tablespoons olive oil
- 1 large can red kidney beans, rinsed and drained
- 1 small chopped red onion
- 1 teaspoon cumin
- Salt, pepper to taste
- 2 c. bread cubes (sur dough is great)
- 1 ½ c. shredded Mozzarella
- 1 tablespoon balsamic vinegar

Serving Size: 4-6

Cooking Time: 45 minutes

zzzzzzzzzzzzzzzzzzzzzzzzzzzzzzzzzzzzzzzzzzzzzzzzzzzzzzzzzzzzzzz

Instructions:

1. Preheat the oven to 375 degrees F.
2. Grease a large rectangular baking dish and set it aside.
3. In a skillet, heat the olive oil and sauté the onion and the fresh spinach for 5 minutes.
4. In a bowl, mix the cooked veggies with the red beans, all the seasonings and the balsamic vinegar.
5. Pour this mixture into the baking dish.
6. Cover with the bread cubes and then the shredded Mozzarella.
7. Bake it in the oven for 35-40 minute or until the cheese is completely melted and golden.

13) Green Tea Squares

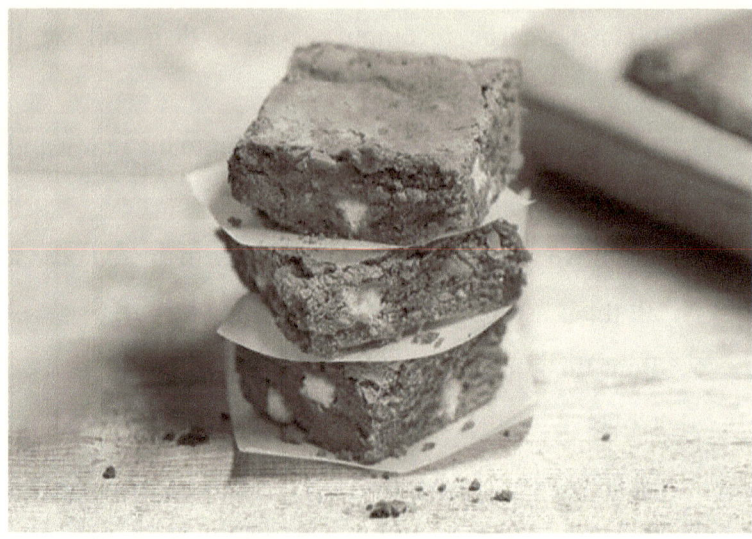

Green tea is served in all coffee shops and restaurants now, and there is a reason behind it. It has been made known that it can seriously help you reduce the aging process of the cells in your body. You can drink it; you can use it as powder form and make some desserts or other soups or dishes. The antioxidants contained in green tea help fight many diseases better as well. So, plenty of reason to incorporate green tea in your regular diet!

Ingredient List:

- 2 c. almond flour
- ½ c. matcha green tea powder
- 2 tablespoons almond milk
- 1 egg
- 1 tablespoon baking powder
- ¼ unsalted butter (room temperature)
- ½ c. brown sugar
- ½ c. dark chocolate chips

Serving Size: 12+

Cooking Time: 45 minutes

zzzzzzzzzzzzzzzzzzzzzzzzzzzzzzzzzzzzzzzzzzzzzzzzzzzzzzzzzzzzzzzzz

Instructions:

1. Preheat oven to 375 degrees F.
2. Prepare square cake pan by spraying non-stick cooking oil.
3. In a large mixing bowl, mix the dry **Ingredient List:** brown sugar, almond flour, baking powder and green tea powder.
4. In a different bowl, mix the butter, egg and almond milk.
5. Combine the dry and wet mixtures and stir until the batter is smooth.
6. Finally, add the chocolate chips and mix again.
7. Pour the batter into the square pan and bake in the oven for 20 to 25 minutes.
8. Remove from the oven, let it cool down, and cut into squares.
9. Store in a cool place until they are all gone!

14) Warm Quinoa Salad with Pomegranate

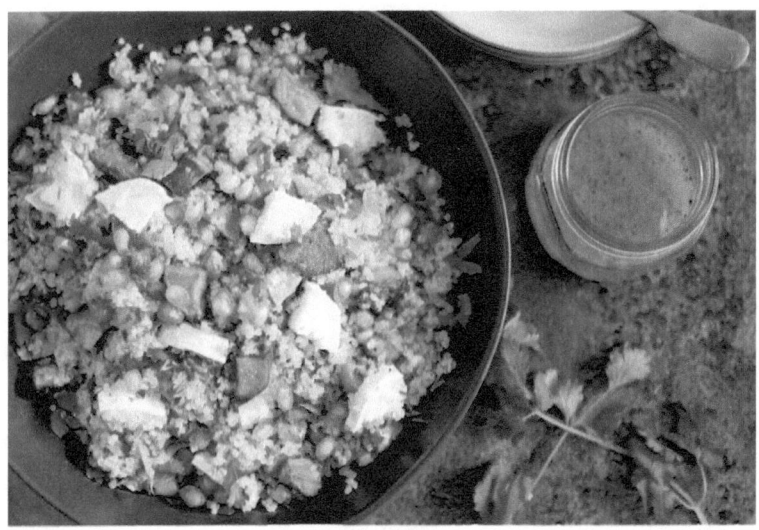

I never used to be very tempted to discover the pomegranate fruit; I think I was intimidated by it. Now that I understand the full health benefits, I definitely try to buy it every chance I get or in season at least. It contains a lot of Vitamin C and antioxidants, helping you once defy that aging process you hate so much. It is very beautiful to serve in many dishes, so go ahead, get out of your comfort zone, and create your next recipe including pomegranate.

Ingredient List:

- 2 c. tricolored uncooked quinoa
- 1 large chopped zucchini
- ½ c. chopped sweet onion
- 4 c. vegetables broth
- 3 tablespoons chopped fresh chives
- 1 c. pomegranate seeds
- 1 c. crumbled feta cheese
- 2 tablespoons lime juice
- 2 tablespoons olive oil
- Salt, pepper to taste
- Smoked paprika
- Sour cream when serving

Serving Size: 4

Cooking Time: 45 minutes

zzzzzzzzzzzzzzzzzzzzzzzzzzzzzzzzzzzzzzzzzzzzzzzzzzzzzzzzzzzzzz

Instructions:

1. Boil 4 cups of vegetables broth and cook the tricolored quinoa as instructed on the package.
2. Meanwhile, use the olive oil to start cooking the sweet onion, fresh chives, and zucchini.
3. Add the lime juice after 10 minutes along with salt and pepper.
4. Once the quinoa is cooked, mix in with the veggies and add the pomegranate seeds, the Feta cheese, and stir well.
5. When it's time to serve, use some sour cream on the side and sprinkle some smoked paprika on top of each serving.

15) Blueberries and More Healthy Popsicles

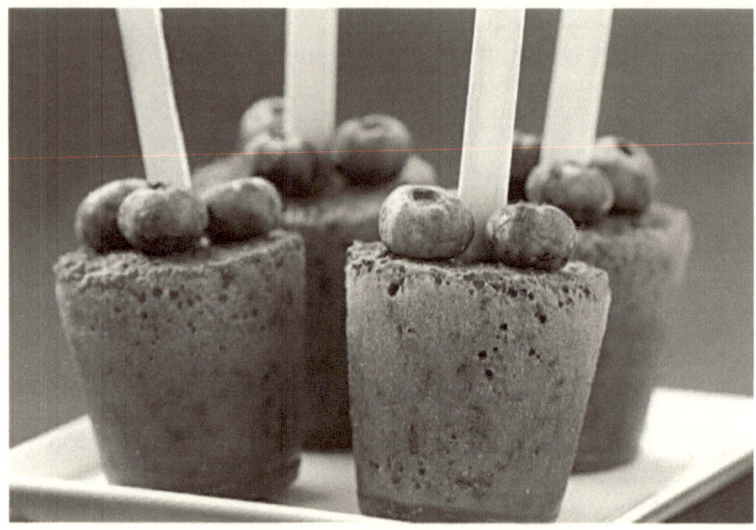

Popsicles usually have an unhealthy connotation. The ones I grew up with anyway were sugary frozen water, and that's it. It does not have to be that way, and you should make an effort as a parent, a spouse, a friend to add many fresh fruits whenever you can. Berries carry antioxidants, helping your skin to stay vibrant and help your body overall be better prepared to fight any infections coming its way.

Ingredient List:

- 1 c. fresh blueberries
- 1 c. fresh raspberries
- Orange juice (about 1 cup)
- Pineapple juice (about 1 cup)
- Lemon juice (about 1 tablespoon)
- 2 Tablespoons honey
- Ice cube trays

Serving Size: 12+

Cooking Time: Few hours

zzzzzzzzzzzzzzzzzzzzzzzzzzzzzzzzzzzzzzzzzzzzzzzzzzzzzzzzzzzzzzz

Instructions:

1. In a bowl, mix the lemon juice, orange juice and honey.
2. In the ice cubes trays, place a little raspberries and blueberries in the bottom of each one.
3. Pour the juice on top until filled up to the top.
4. Freeze for at least an hour.
5. Serve as you go.

16) Savory Oatmeal Lunch

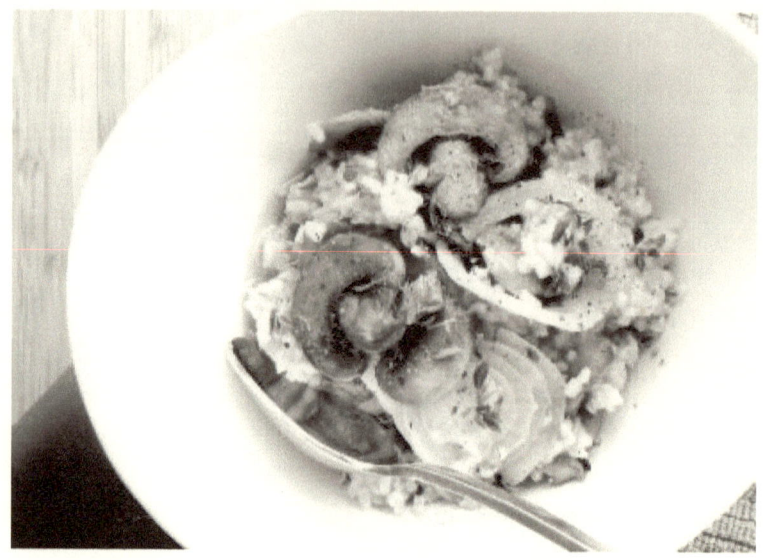

We often run out of ideas on how to prepare oats or oatmeal. Thriving to find new and unique recipes for you every week, I've tackled this challenge. You don't have to serve oats with sweets; this savory recipe is the proof. Oats will provide you some carbs, but low in sugars, meaning your blood sugar can be well controlled. This is directly linked to reducing the acne and wrinkles on your skin. Amazing, right?

Ingredient List:

- 4 c. coconut milk
- 2 c. steel-cut oatmeal
- 2 tablespoons unsalted butter
- 2 c. sliced fresh mushrooms
- 2 minced green onions
- Salt, pepper to taste
- 1 c. shredded pepper jack cheese

Serving Size: 4-6

Cooking Time: 45 minutes

zzzzzzzzzzzzzzzzzzzzzzzzzzzzzzzzzzzzzzzzzzzzzzzzzzzzzzzzzzzzzz

Instructions:

1. Bring to boil the coconut milk on stovetop in a medium pot.
2. Add the oatmeal and lower the temperature; cook until done.
3. Meanwhile, in a medium skillet, sauté the mushrooms, green onions in butter.
4. Season the veggies with salt and pepper.
5. When the oatmeal is done and the veggies are done also, mix them together in the pan.
6. Add the shredded cheese to the mixture and combine well.
7. Keep warm until ready to serve.
8. What a savory way to eat oatmeal!

17) Red Wine Pasta

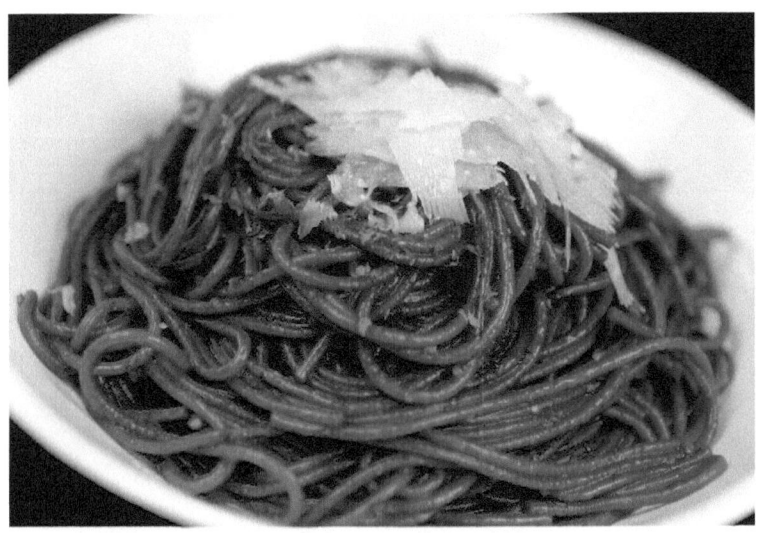

Isn't this great news ladies and gentlemen? Drink up without any guilt. Of course, moderation is the key when it comes to wine, but to know that you can use it to cook or drink an occasional glass of wine and benefit from many properties, is reassuring. That's right, red wine contains an antioxidant name polyphenol and it helps promote DNA repair, so decreasing the process of aging, once again.

Ingredient List:

- 1 box uncooked fettucine
- 1 c. red dry wine
- 3 tablespoons olive oil
- 3 minced cloves garlic
- 2 minced green onions
- 1 c. fresh sliced mushrooms
- 1 chopped green bell pepper
- 2 tablespoons brown sugar
- Pinch cumin
- Salt
- ½ c. shredded Parmesan cheese
- 1 tablespoon red pepper flakes

Serving Size: 4

Cooking Time: 45 minutes

zzzzzzzzzzzzzzzzzzzzzzzzzzzzzzzzzzzzzzzzzzzzzzzzzzzzzzzzzzzzzzz

Instructions:

1. Cook the pasta as indicated on the box or package and set aside.
2. Meanwhile, heat the olive oil, start cooking garlic, onions, mushrooms, bell pepper.
3. When the veggies are cooked, add the red wine, brown sugar, and all seasonings.
4. Add the cooked noodles in the skillet.
5. Sautéed all the ingredients together, adding the Parmesan cheese.
6. Combine well; keep warm until ready to serve.

18) French Baguette and Hardboiled Eggs

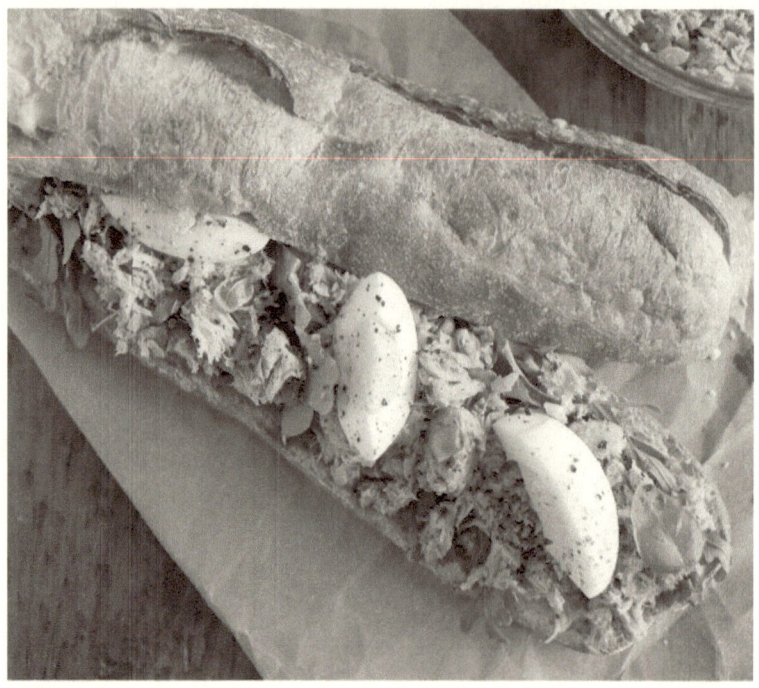

Eggs are relatively cheap to buy but so rich in nutritional value that you must keep eggs in your refrigerator at all times. They are perfect for a last minute meal, omelet, hardboiled eggs and salad or scrambled eggs for breakfast. Eggs will provide you the right amount of nutritional value to help slow your aging process; however, as you probably know already, do not consume raw eggs.

Ingredient List:

- 4 large hardboiled eggs
- 2 c. cooked fresh mixed greens
- 2 cans white tuna in oil, well drained
- 1 tablespoon Dijon mustard
- Salt, pepper to taste
- 1 tablespoon capers
- 4 fresh buttery baguettes

Serving Size: 4

Cooking Time: 45 minutes

ZZZZZZZZZZZZZZZZZZZZZZZZZZZZZZZZZZZZZZZZZZZZZZZZZZZZZZZZZZZZZZ

Instructions:

1. Cut open each baguette, not all the way, and set aside.
2. Spread some Dijon mustard in each of them, and mixed greens, salt, pepper and capers.
3. Finally add a generous portion of tuna and one sliced hardboiled egg.
4. What a nutritious sandwich!

19) Air Fried Eggplant

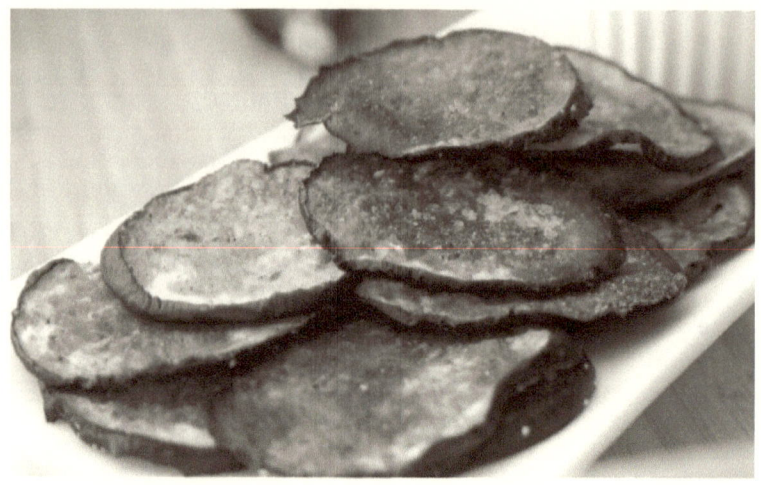

Eggplants are very nutritious. If you are lucky enough to own an air fryer, then there's no reason why you should not prepare them once in a while for your family and friends; it's very tasty. The properties offered by the eggplant are sometimes overlooked. This purple veggie can help improve mental clarity, prevent certain cancers and the amount of antioxidants, just like in a purple food (blueberries), is high and so important for your body.

Ingredient List:

- 1 large eggplant
- 2 egg whites
- 2 c. panko breadcrumbs
- 1 teaspoon garlic powder
- 1 teaspoon onion powder
- Sal, pepper
- ½ c. shredded Swiss cheese
- Cooking oil

Serving Size: 6-8

Cooking Time: 35 minutes

ZZZZZZZZZZZZZZZZZZZZZZZZZZZZZZZZZZZZZZZZZZZZZZZZZZZZZZZZZZ

Instructions:

1. Do not peel the eggplant but slice it in as many ½ inch thick slices as you can.
2. In a large plastic Ziploc type bag place the panko crumbs and all seasonings. Sake it well.
3. Add all the eggplants slices and shake again.
4. In a small bowl, whisk the egg whites and then start dipping each eggplant slice individually.
5. Meanwhile, place the needed oil in your air fryer and cook the eggplant until ready, usually a maximum of 15 minutes or so.
6. Serve with ranch sauce.

20) Turmeric Chicken Stew

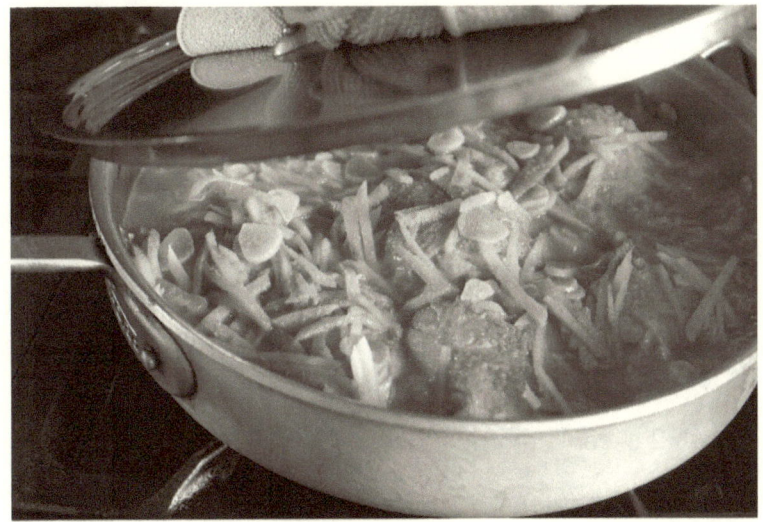

Turmeric is a spice that has a very particular taste and is definitely worth discovering if you haven't yet. It has many amazing properties, include an anti-aging one. This stew is scrumptious, and you can make it with veal or pork if you prefer it to chicken. So, how does turmeric work to keep you young? Just as cinnamon and cloves, its antioxidant content will dramatically help keep your beautiful texture and elasticity to your skin for the years to come.

Ingredient List:

- 2 c. shredded cooked chicken
- 5 c. turkey broth
- 1 c. crushed pineapple
- 2 tablespoons olive oil
- 1 small chopped sweet onion
- 3 minced cloves garlic
- ½ teaspoons turmeric
- Salt, black pepper to taste
- 2 c. cooked brown rice
- 3 tablespoons fresh chopped parsley

Serving Size: 4

Cooking Time: 45 minutes

zzzzzzzzzzzzzzzzzzzzzzzzzzzzzzzzzzzzzzzzzzzzzzzzzzzzzzzzzzzzz

Instructions:

1. In a skillet, heat the oil; cook the sweet onion and garlic.
2. In a saucepan, pour the turkey broth and the crushed pineapple with a little juice.
3. Add all the seasonings. Add the cooked veggies as well.
4. Add the cooked rice and the cooked chicken.
5. Make sure to let it simmer for at least 40 minutes.
6. Taste and adjust the seasonings as needed to your preferences.

21) Stuffed Tomatoes and Cheese

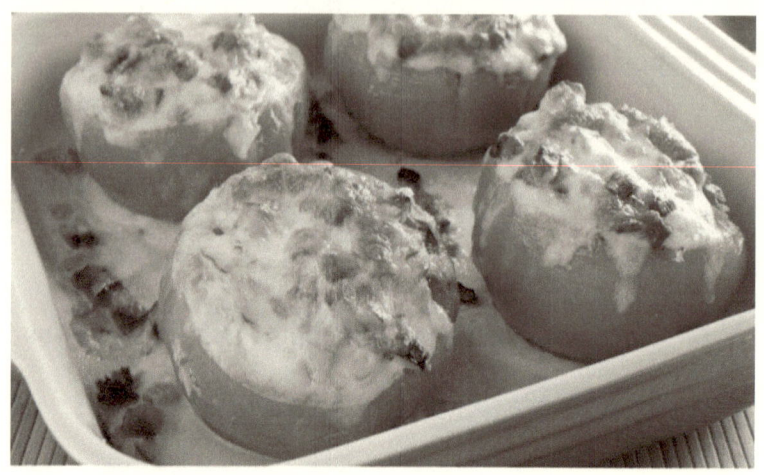

I can eat tomatoes whole, almost like I eat an apple. You can also decide to dress them up and make some stuffed tomatoes for everyone to enjoy. What's important to remember is that this fruit is one of the best anti-aging produce out there: the lycopene found in tomatoes helps to decrease skin damage and helps prevent some serious diseases as well as ensure elasticity and firmness of the skin.

Ingredient List:

- 6 medium tomatoes
- 1 diced avocado
- 2 tablespoons fresh chopped cilantro
- 2 c. ricotta cheese
- 1 c. Seasoned breadcrumbs
- Salt, pepper to taste
- 1 tablespoon garlic powder
- Pinch smoked paprika

Serving Size: 6

Cooking Time: 45 minutes

zzzzzzzzzzzzzzzzzzzzzzzzzzzzzzzzzzzzzzzzzzzzzzzzzzzzzzzzzzzzzzz

Instructions:

1. Preheat oven to 400 degrees F.
2. Prepare all 6 tomatoes by removing the core.
3. In a large mixing bowl, combine the diced avocado, ricotta cheese, breadcrumbs, salt, pepper and garlic powder.
4. Fill each tomato with this mixture.
5. Sprinkle some smoked paprika and chopped cilantro on top of each tomato.
6. Bake in the oven for 30 minutes.

22) Brown Rice with Walnuts

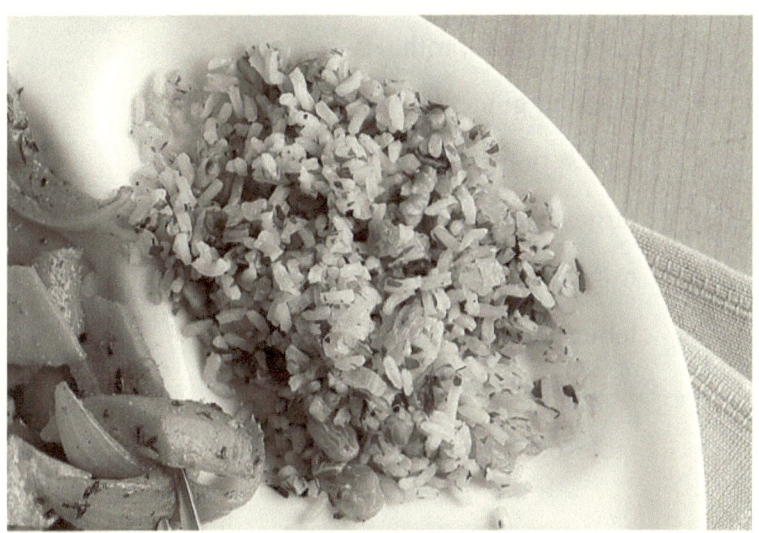

Brown rice should definitely be favored over white rice, all the time. It tastes very good although you might need to get used to it, if you have been a white rice lover for years. It's totally worth it however. Brown rice will give you many extra vitamins, minerals and antioxidants, equipping your body better to fight the process of aging.

Ingredient List:

- 2 c. uncooked brown rice
- 4 c. vegetables broth
- ¼ c. dried golden raisins
- 1 tablespoon walnut oil
- 1 large shredded carrot
- 2 minced cloves garlic
- 1 tablespoon fresh minced ginger
- Salt, pepper to taste
- 1 tablespoon soy sauce

Serving Size: 4

Cooking Time: 45 minutes

zzzzzzzzzzzzzzzzzzzzzzzzzzzzzzzzzzzzzzzzzzzzzzzzzzzzzzzzzzzzzzzz

Instructions:

1. Boil the vegetables broth and cook the brown rice.
2. In a skillet, heat walnut oil, cook the carrot, garlic, fresh ginger.
3. When the rice is done, drain well and transfer into the skillet.
4. Add the soy sauce, salt, pepper and golden raisins.
5. Stir well and keep warm until ready to serve.
6. You can substitute the raisins with dates if you like.

23) Squash and Kale side dish

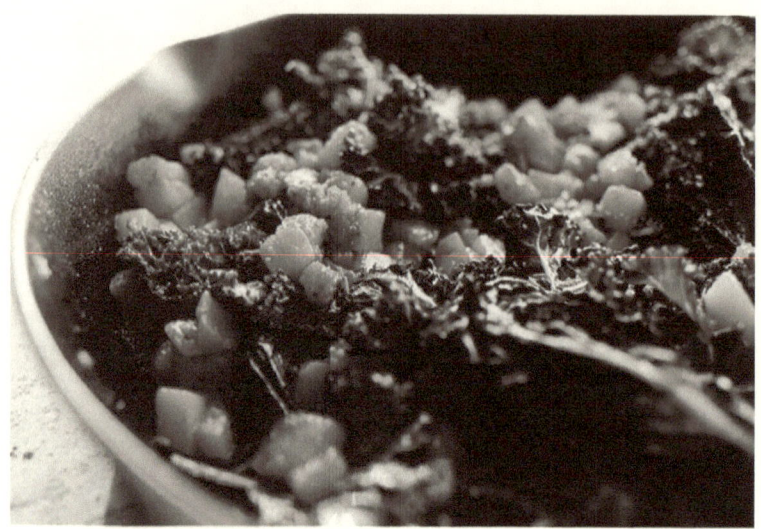

Not only does kale contain very few calories so it is a great food choice when you are on a diet, it also offers many other beneficial properties. It can help reduce inflammation in your body and even arthritis and chronic join pain. Its anti-aging properties are also exceptional, helping your skin to keep looking clear and elastic at the same time.

Ingredient List:

- 1 c. diced prosciutto
- 2 tablespoons olive oil
- Salt, pepper to taste
- 1 tablespoon dried sage
- ½ chopped red onion
- 2 minced cloves garlic
- 4 c. chopped kale leaves
- 2 shredded yellow squash
- 1/3 c. chopped pecans
- 2 tablespoons honey

Serving Size: 4-6

Cooking Time: 50 minutes

zzzzzzzzzzzzzzzzzzzzzzzzzzzzzzzzzzzzzzzzzzzzzzzzzzzzzzzzzz

Instructions:

1. Preheat oven to 400 degrees F.
2. Shred and cut all veggies and prepare all the needed ingredients on the kitchen counter.
3. In a skillet, heat olive oil and cook the garlic, onion, squash and kale for 5 minutes. Set aside.
4. Place all cooked veggies in the bottom of a square greased baking pan.
5. Season with salt, pepper and sage.
6. Sprinkle the diced prosciutto ham on top.
7. Finally, add the chopped pecans and top it off with the honey.
8. Place in the oven and bake for 25 to 40 minutes.

24) Broccoli Slaw Salad

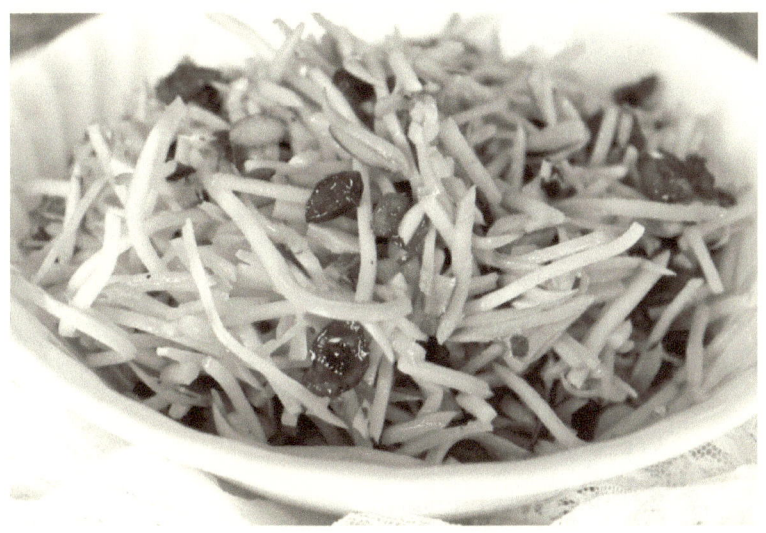

You can purchase broccoli slaw already prepared, ready to mix in with your dressing and other veggies or you can make it from scratch. I honestly prefer to use the pre-shredded starter mix, it makes my life so much easier. The important thing to remember is that it contains so much nutritional value. As far as anti-aging properties, the broccoli can decrease obvious signs of aging, such as wrinkles in your face. Cabbage in general can provide you the same type of value.

Ingredient List:

- 4 c. shredded broccoli or broccoli Cole slaw
- ¼ c. dried cherries
- ½ c. roasted sunflower seed
- ¼ diced red onion
- Dressing
- 2 tablespoons balsamic vinegar
- 2 minced cloves garlic
- ½ teaspoons dry mustard
- ¼ c. olive oil
- 2 tablespoons brown sugar

Serving Size: 4

Cooking Time: 20 minutes

zzzzzzzzzzzzzzzzzzzzzzzzzzzzzzzzzzzzzzzzzzzzzzzzzzzzzzzzzzzzzzzz

Instructions:

1. In a bowl, mix the ingredients for the dressing really well and set aside in the refrigerator for now.
2. In a large bowl, mix the broccoli, the dried cherries, roasted sunflower seeds, and diced red onion.
3. Add the dressing to the salad and mix really well.
4. Divide the mixture in 4 portions.
5. Sometimes I will add some shredded carrots, or shredded red cabbage, if I want to add more color to the salad.

25) Basil and Herb hummus

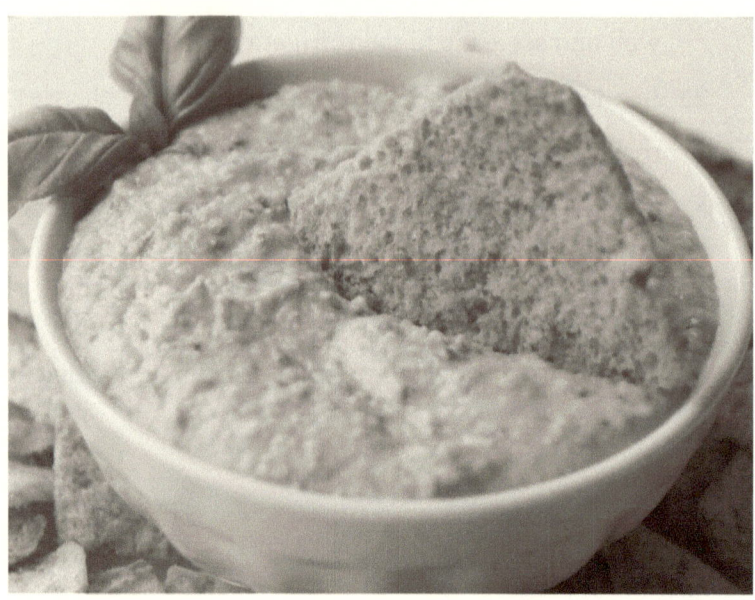

Basil is an awesome herb that can be used in many different types of recipes. It is certainly excellent in tomato sauces, with chicken, and with fish. Try this very unique hummus recipe idea adding basil; you will love the color and the taste. Basil certainly offers great benefits to your body and your skin. Perhaps you have heard of the "holy basil"; basil can help slow down your digestion and also help you decrease your stress level, which is directly linked to a healthier, longer life.

Ingredient List:

- ¼ c. roasted pine nuts
- 2 medium cans chickpeas, rinsed and drained
- 1 c. ½ chopped fresh basil leaves
- 4 minced cloves garlic
- 1/3 c. lime juice
- Salt, black pepper to taste
- ¼ c. sesame oil
- 1 tablespoon sesame seeds
- I tablespoons hot sauce

Serving Size: 4-6

Cooking Time: 45 minutes

zzzzzzzzzzzzzzzzzzzzzzzzzzzzzzzzzzzzzzzzzzzzzzzzzzzzzzzzzzzz

Instructions:

1. After draining the chickpeas well, place them in the food processor.
2. In a skillet, heat oil and cook the garlic and basil leaves.
3. Add in the food processor, the rest of sesame oil, sesame seeds, lime juice salt, pepper and hot sauce.
4. Pulse all these ingredients until very smooth.
5. Add also half of the pine nuts in the mixture. Pulse again.
6. Serve with some nuts and chopped basil on top.

About the Author

A native of Albuquerque, New Mexico, Sophia Freeman found her calling in the culinary arts when she enrolled at the Sante Fe School of Cooking. Freeman decided to take a year after graduation and travel around Europe, sampling the cuisine from small bistros and family owned restaurants from Italy to Portugal. Her bubbly personality and inquisitive nature made her popular with the locals in the villages and when she finished her trip and came home, she had made friends for life in the places she had visited. She also came home with a deeper understanding of European cuisine.

Freeman went to work at one of Albuquerque's 5-star restaurants as a sous-chef and soon worked her way up to head chef. The restaurant began to feature Freeman's original dishes as specials on the menu and soon after, she began to write e-books with her recipes. Sophia's dishes mix local flavours with European inspiration making them irresistible to the diners in her restaurant and the online community.

Freeman's experience in Europe didn't just teach her new ways of cooking, but also unique methods of presentation. Using rich sauces, crisp vegetables and meat cooked to perfection, she creates a stunning display as well as a delectable dish. She has won many local awards for her cuisine and she continues to delight her diners with her culinary masterpieces.

Author's Afterthoughts

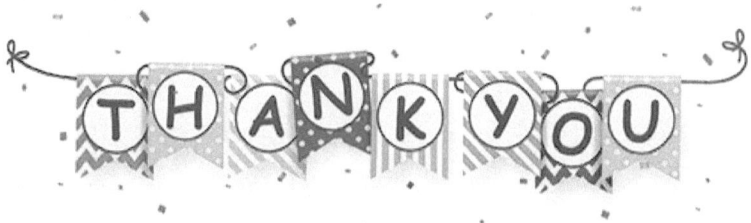

I want to convey my big thanks to all of my readers who have taken the time to read my book. Readers like you make my work so rewarding and I cherish each and every one of you.

Grateful cannot describe how I feel when I know that someone has chosen my work over all of the choices available online. I hope you enjoyed the book as much as I enjoyed writing it.

Feedback from my readers is how I grow and learn as a chef and an author. Please take the time to let me know your thoughts by leaving a review on Amazon so I and your fellow readers can learn from your experience.

My deepest thanks,

Sophia Freeman

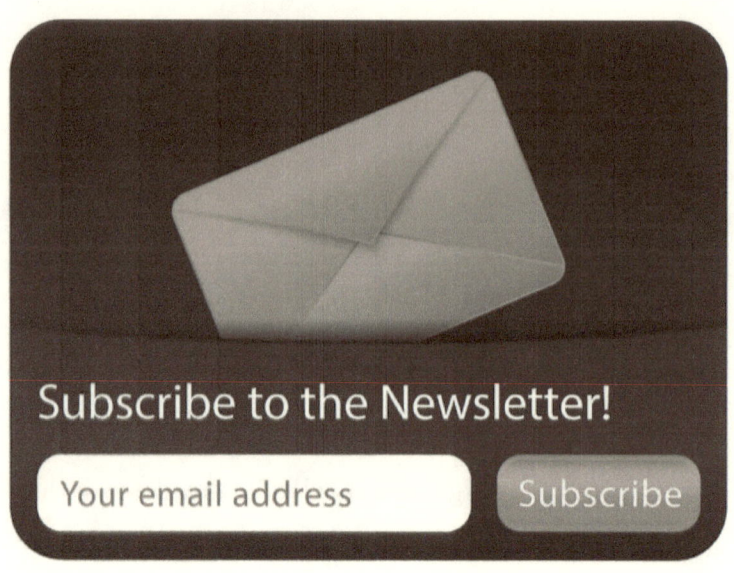

Subscribe to the Newsletter!

Your email address   Subscribe

https://sophia.subscribemenow.com/

★ ★ ★ ★ ★ ★ ★ ★ ★ ★ ★